smokin' cookies

A REAL-LIFE GUIDE TO CONQUERING FOOD ADDICTION AND TRANSFORMING YOUR LIFE

DONNA ELLE

Limits of Liability and Disclaimer of Warranty
The author and publisher shall not be liable for your misuse of this material. This book is strictly for informational and educational purposes. The purpose of this book is to educate and motivate. The author and/or publisher do not guarantee that anyone following these techniques, suggestions, tips, ideas, or strategies will become successful. The author and/or publisher shall have neither liability no responsibility to anyone with respect to any loss or damage caused, or alleged to be caused, directly or indirectly by the information contained in this book.
Views expressed in this publication do not necessarily reflect the views of the publisher.

Cover design by Eric Finley
Editing by Keen Vision Editing, LLC

Printed in the United States of America
ISBN 978-1-941749-46-3
4-P Publishing
Chattanooga, TN 37411

Contact Donna

If you would like Donna to speak at your next event, contact her at the following:

E-Mail - donna@donnaellewellness.com

Website -www.donnaellewellness.com

FB - www.facebook.com/Donnas-D.I.V.A.s

Join Donna's mailing list to receive monthly motivational tips to help you stay successful on your journey to the new you.

www.donnaellewellness.com

WHAT D.I.V.A.S ARE SAYING...

It's the beginning of a new year and I've decided to share something I've never really shared before, mostly with the hopes I can help motivate someone to do the same in 2014. With the new year comes new goals and resolutions. Losing weight is always on the top of that list.

Everyone who is truly motivated has or will have that moment when, for lack of better words, it just clicks. Some viewers have asked me when my moment was. I lost 30 pounds in 2013 but my turning point/aha moment happened in summer 2012 at a Nightfall concert.

Van Hunt (if you don't know who he is Google him...it's worth it) performed in Chattanooga. After the concert I was lucky and bold enough to introduce myself and get a picture. Yes, I was that girl...after I took my picture with Mr. Hunt I was extremely excited to tweet it, post it on Facebook, and tell the world I'd just met one of my favorite artists. I took my phone and smiling looked down at it. I paused and tears welled up in my eyes. I didn't recognize the person in the picture.

"Look at those arms," I thought. "When did my face get so round?" I never shared that picture with anyone but a few close friends...until now. People tell me, "I didn't realize you were that...big". Well, I was and if I stopped taking care of myself I could be again.

The moment I saw that picture and allowed myself to really take it in, no need for denial, was the moment that changed how I lived in the Scenic City. The very next day I was watching what I put in my mouth and in the gym more often.

Fast forward to winter, 2012. I joined a sisterhood like no other. At first Classes were painful and excruciatingly difficult. I was sore for days and dreaded working that hard ever again. In high school I trained as an athlete but that was a decade ago and my body just isn't the same.

However, I knew I wouldn't...I couldn't quit. I was, after all, one of the youngest members of the group and if these 30, 40 and 50 something-year-olds could do it than I sure as hell could. For two days a week I stuck with it. As time passed I began to notice the change in my body, my attitude and my energy. I feel like an athlete again and this is just the beginning.

This winter marked my one-year anniversary with Donna and the D.I.V.A.s. I have changed but I have also watched their physiques transform. These women have helped motivate me to perform my best and keep going, no matter what. I'm truly grateful to be a part of such a wonderful team. That's what it is, a team.

I continue to struggle sometimes but I haven't completely fallen off the wagon, nor will I. This year I'm determined to look and feel my very best, I'm not done yet. I've learned not to take my strength for granted and instead use it to help those who may need an extra push to become their best.

Jonquil

DEDICATION

To my mother and son who have been my source of encouragement throughout my weight loss journey. I am eternally grateful to you both.

ABOUT THE AUTHOR

Donna Elle can say with conviction she has been called to help others realize their personal worth and invest in themselves. With more than 20 years of experience in the public eye as a radio host and television personality, Donna Elle has reached out to and helped people from all walks of life. Donna has been driven to succeed since childhood. At the age of 13 she became a teen reporter for WJTT, Power 94 in Chattanooga. For the next six years, Donna focused on her talent for radio and at the age of 19, she was hired as a full-time radio personality. After 22 years on air, she decided to pursue another dream– a career in television. In 2012, Donna joined the Eyewitness News Team at WRCB-TV in Chattanooga as a reporter, photographer, editor, and television host. She also was the midday personality for iheartradio.

While her dreams are coming to fruition, she has not forgotten about her mission to inspire. Ten years ago, Donna worked hard to achieve a goal that she is very proud of. With eating in moderation, a supportive group of friends and family, and exercise regimen, she has lost over ninety pounds. Donna made the decision to help women like her, and teach them to invest in themselves and while taking their health seriously.

Donna is the CEO and Founder of Donna Elle Wellness and Donna's D.I.V.A.s Workout Classes. In 2011, Donna was featured in Ebony Magazine for her accomplishments with weight loss. She also empowers through motivational speaking, Healthy Lifestyle Coaching and teaching

D.I.V.A.s classes for women at all levels of fitness. Donna's D.I.V.A.s. (Determined Individuals Valuing

Activities) with a goal to get 100,000 everyday women off the couch and start moving for a lifetime!"

Donna's purpose is to bring out the best in people regardless of circumstance. Her proudest accomplishment is raising her son Brandon who is now a college student. Donna is a mother, career woman, and motivator that has a heart for people. Her personal motto is… *"Invest in you today…Live tomorrow"*

CONTENTS

INTRODUCTION

Would you like to know what I hate? I hate it when people who have never had a weight problem write books that give unrealistic dreams and hopes about weight loss. Luckily for you, this is not that kind of book!

First things first, allow me to introduce myself. My name is Donna Elle. If you're in the Chattanooga, TN area, you may recognize my name from radio or television. If not, then don't worry. You'll soon learn who I am. You see, I'm on a mission. I'm on a journey to empower women of every race, color, size, marital status, hair type, and complexion; every woman who has a dream or desire to be better; every woman who felt afraid to look in the mirror; every woman who felt like she was alone with no one to share her sorrows. For over twenty years, food was my addiction. I felt so alone on my journey to lose weight. I can't count the number of times I felt like throwing in the towel, but because of you, her, her, and her, I didn't. I made a promise to myself (and someone very special to me) that once I reached the promise land (my ideal weight) I would come back to get as many women as I could.

Before I attempt to tell you how to fix your business, let me continue to tell you mine. I've been a part of the local media since I was 13 years old. I started as a teen reporter on Power 94 here in Chattanooga, TN. I am the mother of one handsome, young man and a friend to many. Most beneficial to you and the purpose of this book, I'm a former fat girl who has changed her life to LIVE better! I know, fat is such a tough word. I'll admit, it stings a bit to even say it from time to time. I have no problem using the term 'fat' because it describes who I used to be. It describes who I return to at some moments. To me, being a 'fat' girl has nothing to do with actual weight. "Fat" has everything to do with your diet – what you eat! You can be a nice size five and still have a 'fat' eating style or a "fat way of living"!

For the past seven years, I've taught aerobics, circuit training, and boot camp classes. I'm not just an exercise instructor and former fat girl. I motivate people to lose weight, learn to be confident in their own skin, live a healthier lifestyle, and live life to the fullest! As an AFFA certified instructor, my goal is to help people feel amazing about who they are, not who they are going to become. It's not just about their weight. My aim is to help every woman I come in contact with feel better about who she is mentally, physically, and spiritually.

Sounds simple enough, right? I know what you're thinking. This woman got up one day, decided to lose weight, and BAM! Just like that it happened. I worked out every day, ate green veggies, and drank water until it ran from my nose – and did it all with a smile. Right? Wrong! Brace yourself. I'm about to give you a little insight into the real-life struggles of a fat girl.

The primary focus of this book is to discuss realistic ways to meet your weight-loss goals, but it's more than that. The inspiration found among these pages can be applied to any area of life. This book is not just for women who are overweight, *Smoking Cookies* serves as a guide for any woman who desires a change.

Regardless of what size you are, it's time to take control of who you are by changing your mind, which will in turn change your actions. It all starts with simply devoting an hour a day to yourself. *Smoking Cookies* will show you ways to build your self-esteem and productivity through repetition.

We lose many things along our journey through life, but one of the hardest things to lose is weight. Sometimes, we as women get so caught up in the day to day bustle of life that we let ourselves go. Somewhere in between caring for everyone else (or somebody else, for my single and divorced women) we lose ourselves; we lose our hope, and we lose our ambition. I challenge you, right now, to begin happening to life, and stop allowing life to happen to you! Take control! Life is not meant to be run on autopilot. I challenge you to take the necessary steps to regain who you truly are. You do not have to accept weight gain, unhealthy living, and mediocrity as a way of life. What do you want for yourself?

Regardless of where you are in life, I'm going to help you find that inspiration you need to get off the couch and chase the lifestyle you want. If you want to feel good about yourself, preserve your life span, or be active with your children or grandchildren, I'm going to help you get there! I hear what you're saying:

"Donna, you don't understand, girl. I got these kids running everywhere!"

"Donna, I have class every morning and I work at night."

"Donna, my husband and these kids take up all my time."

"Donna, I've tried so many weight loss programs. They never work."

"Donna, my schedule won't allow it!"

"But, Donna, what about my hair?"

Blah, blah, blah! So what! Again, I'm a motivator and fitness instructor. So I've heard it all before! The time for making excuses ended the moment you picked up this book! Now is the time to take a few moments out of the day to work on becoming a better you! It doesn't matter if you've tried multiple diets in the past. It's okay if you fell off the wagon and you are having a hard time getting back on. Stop wallowing in your past failures. It's time to become the change you want to see! My vow is to help you get there! Before you begin using this book, I want you to ask yourself two questions:

1.) How will you feel once you take this step?
2.) How will you feel if you don't take this step?

Whatever your answers are, write them down. Tape it up somewhere in your house, car, work, or wherever! Put it in your phone or iPad! Keep your reasons in plain view so that when the going gets a little tough, you'll be motivated to keep pushing!

Each chapter offers a brief story of the obstacles I encountered along my weight loss journey. At the end of each chapter, you'll find what I like to refer to as "Cookie Bites". So many times, we talk about what we want to do, but never take the necessary actions to actually do what we want to do. Cookie Bites are small steps to help you on your journey to conquering food addiction. Each question is designed to make you think about your current situation and identify answers that will assist you on your journey.

Enough of the small talk, are you ready? Take a deep breath!

LET'S GOOOOO D.I.V.A.S!

COOKIE CONTRACT

L ife happens. I get it! Sometimes, situations like death, job loss, family drama, unexpected life changes, finances, and stress cause us to get sidetracked from what we truly desire. Those things are a part of LIFE and we have to learn how to sift through. We can do it! There comes a time where you have to decide what is a priority, what is just a distraction, or what can you maneuver through. All tests are designed to strengthen us, but sometimes the enemy attempts to make us believe that our situations are our final destinations. So not true! I declare right now that you will not be distracted, and you will have the victory! Despite every obstacle that has been thrown or will be thrown, you will make the necessary actions to improve your lifestyle! Now it's time to sign your name on the dotted line! That's right! We're about to make this thing official. **The Cookie Contract** is between you and your dream to be better! **The Cookie Contract** binds you to your aspirations. In the court of law, you will be the judge, juror, lawyer, and defendant.

You can choose a life sentence of well-being, or a life sentence of excuses and unhealthiness. The choice is up to you! This contract is for you, for us! By signing this contract, you vow to become a priority, to focus on things of value, to remain positive, and to become the healthiest, most confident you for YOU. Feel free to involve your friends, a team, church, some D.I.V.A.s, or even family. Don't fill it out immediately. Remember, contracts are binding!! Take some time alone to meditate on your answers. You must complete **The Cookie Contract** before continuing *Smoking Cookies.*

Appoint your spouse, child, best friend, or even your mom as a witness to help hold you accountable. You are worth it!

THE COOKIE CONTRACT

I,_____, agree to make steps to be healthy for a lifetime. I am worth this journey! When I put myself first, I will become powerful, successful, and LIVE my best life. I know being healthy isn't solely about what's on the scale, but also how I feel about myself. I deserve to make permanent changes. I owe myself a new, healthy diet and exercise routine. My goal is to make healthier choices and eat what I enjoy in moderation. I can conquer this addiction!

I will forgive myself for past mistakes. I will fight for the future I deserve. I will conquer today and focus consistently on my goals for tomorrow. I am worth it! I will no longer make excuses for not working out. I will work hard to make better choices. If I fail, I know tomorrow is a new day. I will no longer attempt to justify unhealthy behaviors. I understand that I am not perfect. I will not miss out on opportunities to be active and live! I will make this choice for me and allow others to reap the benefits. I will be the best me!

I know that I can reach my small term and long term goals by developing a new mindset and new healthy habits. I am worth it! I have the power to change my relationship with myself, my surroundings, food, or any other addictions I may have. I can and will reach my goal step by step, day by day. I am worth it!

Date_____

Signature_____

Witness_____

WE WERE MADE FOR EACH OTHER

"Life expectancy would grow by leaps and bounds if green vegetables smelled as good as bacon," ~ Doug Larson

Even though she was a single parent, my mother was amazing! She took care of my sister and me, motivated us, and constantly believed in us. My mom is my rock. My grandmother meant the world to me as well. She played a big role in helping my mother raise us. I didn't meet my father until my 23rd birthday. As a child, I often thought about him. Now that I'm older, I realize that I often sought validation from people because of his absence. This caused me to "reach out" to people and food and feel empty more than I should have, but that's another story for another day! I'm ready to talk about what was once my favorite subject, food!

All addictions start from somewhere. While you may indulge in your addiction when you get stressed or depressed, it doesn't start there. If we are ever to get rid of our addictions, we must first locate the root, where it all began. For me, my addiction was food! This food addiction started when I was a just a little girl.

First of all, my family loves food! When we celebrate, we eat. When we are stressed, we eat. When we have a family gathering, we eat. My family always looked forward to a good meal! So being a little chunky was okay. Growing up, my grandmother was never bothered by my weight. She knew I loved a good meal. Let's just say that didn't make it easier! That woman could throw down in the kitchen! Ironically enough, my grandmother was not overweight. Her main objective was always to feed her friends and family; she did an amazing job. Each holiday she would cook for the entire family (five children and a gazillion grandkids). She also had club meetings where she would cook for her closest friends. I'm still wondering what those meetings were about! At the time, however, I didn't care! All I knew was her friends were coming over, and I would have FOOD! She would make so much food for everybody, but the funny thing is, I never saw her eat! As I got older, I realized that cooking was her way of showing us how much she loved us.

> If we are ever to get rid of our addictions, we must first locate the root, where it all began.

I remember how my grandmother would make me breakfast in the morning before school. It would be so good! I can still envision those tender, juicy, slices of country ham lying on a bed of fluffy, white, buttered rice along with soft, homemade biscuits and red eye gravy. She had no problem waking me up for school in the morning. One whiff of her cooking was enough to make me hop right out of bed and shoot straight to the kitchen table. When she picked me up after school, she always had a little 'snack' for me. This little 'snack' (as she would call it) consisted of whatever was left after breakfast. It was never just a bite or two. It was always the same amount I'd eaten earlier, if not more. This was something she gave me just to tide me over until dinner. Get this. As a child, I hated washing dishes. It's not exactly my favorite thing to do as an adult either. On Sundays, I would always look forward to my grandmother's big, Sunday dinners. However, the dishes that accumulated in the midst of her cooking and serving also made me dread Sundays. But, of course, me being the fat kid that I was, I found a way to see the "sweeter side" of things. I realized that if I did the dishes, I would have the opportunity to sneak a few more bites of my grandmother's homemade cobbler. I was strategic when it came to getting food. After everyone finished eating, I would jump to the sink to begin washing the dishes. As soon as everyone got settled in the living room, I would walk very softly to the stove, slowly open it, and move my spoon in for the kill! Smacking on those huge spoonfuls of cobbler made washing the dishes a lot of fun!

As for my mother, she believed that I had so much potential. She desired for me to be more than just a pretty face. My mother wanted me to be healthy and active. She wanted me to be able to go outside and run around like other children my age. My mom kept me active growing up with my family. While my mother knew that kids teased me sometimes, she didn't know how bad it was. My mom did the best she could at the time. She was a single parent of two girls. She didn't realize how mean children could be to children who were different.

As a little girl, I never wanted to work out, run, race, or do anything that required me to sweat or move around for long periods of time. But my mom constantly encouraged me to, she was always active. Whenever someone would throw a ball, I'd move to avoid having to catch it. That was just not my thing. Whenever kids gathered to play a game outside, I'd get lost so that I wouldn't have to play. For one, I

> I was strategic when it came to getting food... Smacking on those huge spoonfuls of cobbler made washing the dishes a lot of fun!

was way too prissy for all of that sweating nonsense. My mother kept me dressed so pretty – bows and ribbons everywhere. I didn't want to get dirty. Would you believe I didn't get a scratch on my legs until I was a teenager?

Secondly, I wasn't as fast as other kids, and I knew it. Whenever I tried to be active, the kids would joke and tease me. Sometimes, it felt like they just couldn't wait to watch me plop down on the grass to catch my breath. They never missed an opportunity to tease the fat, chubby girl. I caught it everywhere – on the playground, in the neighborhood, in the classroom, and even on field trips. Their all-time favorite joke was: "Hey, you want some candy?" Each time I would say yes, and each time, they would burst into laughter. They never actually had any candy to give me. They just got a kick out of hearing the fat girl say she wanted something to eat.

It didn't take me long to realize that I was different from my peers. At home, being a little overweight was okay. My family would say things like, "You were the heaviest baby to carry!" as if it were a badge of honor or something. Again, cooking was the love language that my family responded to, so naturally, having a little extra 'loving' here and there was normal. At school, it was totally different. The kids were a lot smaller and way more active. It was hard for my family to understand that people didn't choose me for activities. No one wanted to pick the fat girl to be on their team for kickball or softball. It didn't matter that I was always dressed in the nicest clothes. That just made me a fat girl in a pretty dress. My weight made me an easy target.

The teasing only got worse as I got older. Shortly after middle school, I began to make peace with my weight and my love for food. Don't get me wrong, it still hurt when people joked about my weight. I felt like I was the only one in the world being teased. Whenever they would joke and laugh about my weight, it seemed like everyone could hear them. Teasing began to play on my mentality. Whenever I went somewhere, I felt like everyone was staring, pointing, and laughing at me. My mind began to tell me that people only saw my weight.

As a way to retaliate, I started to joke back! My response to the teasing became, "Hey, I can change my body, but you can't change your face." People would laugh. Sure, it was funny for a moment. But pretty soon, even that wore off, and I was back to being teased again. I still had to live with the humiliation of being teased. This humiliation only led me draw closer to the one thing that never let me down – food! So I decided to make a difference! I fell in love with Oprah and decided I wanted to be just like her. Everyone loved Oprah. I desired that same attention. I became outspoken in order to take the attention off of me. I broke out of my shy shell and became an extrovert. I started singing in 3rd grade, participating in plays, and writing music. My objective was to prove everyone else wrong. My dream was to become a star!

Of course, my family didn't mean any harm. In fact, most families suffer from the same problem. Back in the day, food wasn't as easy to acquire as it is now. Even in certain parts of the world, like Africa, being a little plump is a sign of wealth! It's not easy to break generational traditions. I'll tell you first hand, it has not been easy for me and my family. To break habits and addictions, we must be intentional in all of our actions. For my mother and I, we found different ways to be active. At family gatherings, family vacations we hold each other accountable for limiting our intake of unhealthy food. Our focus was moderation and not elimination. We also wanted to try the goodies. Can you imagine being around so many delicious dishes and having to eat it in moderation? It was rough, but it has been well worth it!

> My objective was to prove everyone else wrong. My dream was to become a star!

Most think that people are fat just because the food is good. That is only partially true. There are root issues that drive you towards any addiction. Remember my emptiness longing for validation. That led to my emotional eating. You know how there's an All Addicts Anonymous (AAA) group? Well, I created my AAA to fight addictions.

Acknowledge, Address, and Act

➤ **Acknowledge** that you have an addiction. Be real with yourself. What do you run to when you are down and out? Is it healthy?

➤ **Address** it. Instead of charging into your problem head first, find out where it comes from. Addictions are just like trees. You can trim the branches, but if you don't treat the roots, you will continuously run into the same problems. What's the address of your addiction? Does it reside in your childhood? A traumatic life experience?

➤ **Act** on it. Create a simple, reasonable plan to rid yourself of your addiction. So many times we create elaborate plans to do better, only to get overwhelmed and disappointed. Again, be real with yourself. What can you do right where you are? Start there and climb higher. Don't just run to the top of the ladder only to get tired and climb back down. Take it in strides and reward yourself at each step.

COOKIE BITES

1. Why do you overeat? How does it make you feel?

2. What emotions are most likely to trigger you to indulge in your addiction?

3. What actions could you take to replace that emotion?

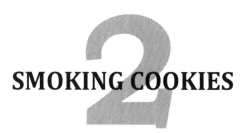

SMOKING COOKIES

"Some people drink alcohol, some smoke cigarettes, but I used to smoke a pack of cookies every night!" ~ Donna Elle

S o let's talk a little bit about my infatuation with food. As a little girl, food became my best friend. I didn't need anyone to talk to me during recess. I had enough honey buns and cookies crammed in my book bag to keep me company for hours. I had even begun to make myself believe that having more snacks than the other kids would make them jealous of me. "Nah, nah, nah, nah, nah! I got some snacks!" I would say. The sad thing was no one heard me. They were too busy laughing or running around having fun. Food was "my love", my best friend. Most girls were excited about seeing their crush at school (I was too), but I was more excited about all the snacks and treats I packed in my book bag to enjoy. Food gave me a sense of peace that nothing else could provide. Don't get me wrong, I had friends. But I was always wondering what they thought of me. I wondered if they thought I was the "fat friend" in the group. Did they make fat jokes behind my back? The thoughts in my head often made me shy away from them. Luckily for me, I had food. Food never let me down. It never dropped me. It never judged me. It never had an opinion of me. I never had to worry about food talking behind my back. I could trust food to make me feel better no matter what happened. Food was my ride or die!

Of course being overweight led to other problems. As a child, I wanted so dearly to be accepted. I wanted people to see me, to see Donna, but for a while, I believed no one did. Whenever I did find any meaningful friendships, I did all I could to keep them. Even if it meant to be used or let down. I was afraid of being rejected. I had a fear of losing people. Once I began dating, I worried about being accepted as an overweight woman. I would go to a restaurant with a guy and try to eat very little. I didn't even enjoy the date because I was so busy worried about how I was eating! I never wanted to come in first place in the "food finish". In the back of my mind, I didn't want to be the stereotypical fat girl who ordered five entrees and cleaned each plate! I would order something small and cute like a salad only to devour everything in the kitchen once I got home. Being teased conditioned me to be empty. Food would always be there to welcome me with open arms.

> Food gave me a sense of peace that nothing else could provide... I could trust food to make me feel better no matter what happened. Food was my ride or die!

Whenever I got stressed, I would eat something every ten minutes. Living two minutes away from a gas station didn't make it any better. Sometimes, I would buy M&Ms to take home, but by the time I got from one traffic light to the next, the whole bag would be gone! At that moment, I would feel so satisfied. I had this sick sense of accomplishment, but the next day I would feel so bad about who I was. It depressed me. I felt tired and exhausted. The only thing that made me happy again was more food!

Food was comfort for me. One of my favorite restaurants was Red Lobster. I would have crab legs, the Admiral's Feast (that came with shrimp, scallops, clams, a baked potato, and salad), at least six cheddar bay biscuits, and a slice of chocolate cake. I would gobble down all of my food and wait patiently for my son to finish his plate; praying that he wouldn't eat all of it so that I could! I began to stop caring about what people thought of my eating habits. I held my head up high when I ordered my four apple pies. I smiled brightly as I reached for my son's plate to finish whatever he left. Food brought me so much joy. Being without food felt lonely. Sure, it was pretty embarrassing to be in public cleaning up plates like a garbage disposal, but my relationship with food trumped everything. I told myself I needed those apple pies, better yet I deserved those apple pies for all of the meanies and teasing I had endured. I

> ...in the privacy of my home, I'd smoke row after row of whatever I could get my hands on. Cookies, cakes, and candy. It didn't matter! As long as it was sweets, it was getting smoked. That was my drug of choice.

figured that after all I'd been through, the least life could give me was a little time with my best friend – food.

Hello, I'm Donna, and I'm Addicted to FOOD!

When people do drugs, I mean really do drugs, they do them in private. Serious drug users don't need a crowd. They don't need a group of people with them to get their high. They don't get high where the world can see. Drug addicts prefer to be alone. At that moment, they are satisfied and at peace because they think no one is looking at them. I should know. I've never been addicted to heroin, cigarettes, or alcohol, but I was addicted to food. I didn't like to eat in public because I was afraid that people would judge me. Oh, but in the privacy of my home, I'd smoke row after row of whatever I could get my hands on.

> My life became unmanageable because I put so much into feeding my addiction and it was hard to focus on making my other goals a reality.

Cookies, cakes, and candy. It didn't matter! As long as it was sweets, it was getting smoked. That was my drug of choice.

Whenever I was stressed out, I would go to the store for cookies. I'm not talking about the cute little six-packs; I would buy one of those super packs with almost 100 cookies in them. When I got home, my son would look at me with his hands out-stretched. I'd reluctantly pull out three of the cookies to give him. I didn't even sit down to enjoy the cookies. I would stand in the kitchen to eat them because I didn't want him to see me eating the rest of the cookies for two reasons. Reason number one, I was embarrassed. Reason number two, I didn't want him to ask for another one! My life became unmanageable because I put so much into feeding my addiction and it was hard to focus on making my other goals a reality. It had reached the point where the only thing I looked forward to was a good meal or sweets. My primary goal became getting my next meal or cookie. This goal was attainable because all I had to do was buy it. I did it all the time and, therefore, knew it was possible. Everything else seemed like a pipe dream. I could go to a restaurant be mentally satisfied because I told myself that it calmed my nerves. Therefore, in my mind, that's exactly what it did. I couldn't focus on anything else. I was a slave to food.

When I got my hands on something sweet, it would "trigger "me to eat unhealthy for the rest of my day! I realized that I couldn't bring my triggers in the house.

I know what you're thinking, you have kids and family members that might sneak your triggers in. Here's where you bring the entire family together to help you with your weight loss goals. Make sure everyone knows that you can't have (whatever your trigger is). Make a team effort to get healthy for life!

It's unfair how most addictions are easily hidden, but if you are overweight the world knows your problem! We can change that! I am not asking you to deprive yourself. I am asking you to limit yourself. Ask your mate to put your triggers in a place where you won't see it daily. Try not to buy your triggers in large quantities. It's all about eating in moderation! Some of the questions that I ask my girls to ask themselves are, what do you feel when you're eating? What is that emotion? What's your motivation to stay healthy? These questions are necessary to help you avoid overcompensating your triggers.

COOKIE BITES

What are your trigger foods? For me, it was cookies or sweets.

1. What are your trigger foods?

2. Are you addicted to food or are you an overeater?

3. What is your favorite meal? Is it Unhealthy?

4. What could you do to replace your food addiction?

5. What day of the week would you like to have a small treat meal or dessert?

WHEN THE COOKIE CRUMBLES

"You can't lose weight by talking about it. You have to keep your mouth shut." ~Unknown

I will never forget the day I decided get off the couch and make a change! It was Labor Day, so you can imagine how it went down. There I was, overweight, sitting at the table with a mountain of food so high you could barely see my face (which was fine by me). My plate was sitting right! I had two hot dogs loaded with all the fixings, a helping of baked beans and a mound of ribs with barbeque sauce dripping from the sides like a mini volcano. As other family members ran around with each other having fun, I sat and had a little fun of my own. I ate and ate and ate until I made myself sick. I'm sure after the two hot dogs, I wasn't even hungry anymore, but it didn't matter. My addiction to food was so surreal that eating was like sport to me. If someone had created a food-eating team, I'd be well qualified, well trained, and ready to sign up! I went to the restroom and on my way out, I caught a glimpse of myself in the mirror. I looked at myself for a while as I rubbed my aching belly. I was disgusted with what I saw. Most importantly how I felt! Why on earth had I eaten so much? I made up my mind right at that moment that enough was enough. It was time to lose weight.

Like so many, I yo-yo dieted for years. I was on my first diet when I was fourteen years old. It wasn't until I turned twenty-nine that I decided to change my life for good. From age fourteen to twenty-nine, I experienced a series of ups and downs that made it hard for me to commit to losing weight. I didn't have any real goals for my health. I was confident in my career. I had seen myself one way for so long it was becoming difficult to see past it. At the age of twenty-nine, I re-evaluated myself and opted for longevity instead of the yo-yo that had kept me from reaching my goals. At twenty-nine, I had been a mom for almost ten years. In addition to my desire to feel better about who I was, I became conscious of how my son saw me. This realization helped me to finally get serious about losing weight.

> I was disgusted with what I saw. Most importantly how I felt! Why on earth had I eaten so much? I made up my mind right at that moment that enough was enough. It was time to lose weight.

I began by working out with my mom. I would sporadically take an aerobics class with her. Aerobics class was fun! As a big girl, I knew I had something to prove. Those skinny girls thought they would out-do me. Boy, they had another think coming! Would you believe I got in front of the group for the entire class just to prove that I could keep up with them?

Since I was a little girl, I was always on someone's stage in the public eye. People watched me, and I didn't mind. I found peace on stage; it was just what I wanted. I had dreams of becoming as famous as Oprah! I looked up to her as a child. I imagined myself being on every television in every home across the nation. Instead of the fat Donna I saw when I looked in the mirror, I would be the awesome Donna, who everyone loved and adored.

In public, I was the "Baddest Big Girl" in this city. That's right, I said it. The "Baddest Big Girl" in Chattanooga and would defend my crown if I had one. People knew me as the beautiful big girl who always dressed nice! In public, I'd smile and exude D.I.V.A.! I'd be that Donna everyone heard on the radio. But it was all just a façade. All they saw was a beautiful smile and a bunch of confidence, but what they didn't see was the desire to be accepted. The desire to be loved despite my food addictions and despite my weight. Sometimes, I wore a smile to avoid crying or wanting just to run away and hide.

I got so many compliments that went something like this, "Oh, you have the prettiest face. Or, "Girl, you know how to dress!" To me, all I heard was, "You're cute, and you can dress, but your body is gone to hell."

At my maximum weight, I weighed four pounds shy of 300. I knew I didn't quite have a banging Halle Berry body, but dang! Big girls need a little love too! I desired to hear compliments about my shape and my true personality.

Starting a workout routine was a pretty easy step for me. It gave me a stage to perform on and nothing could beat my sense of accomplishment as I successfully finished each aerobics class while girls one-third of my size were complaining two minutes in. Though this part was fairly simple, the journey was far from it. It became a lot harder than I thought it would be.

After a while, the honeymoon phase was over. You see, newlyweds aren't the only people who experience honeymoons. The honeymoon phase is usually the result of something inspiring. When you overcome the desire to sit when you don't feel like moving you'll notice that you may get the feeling of, "Hey, this is easy." But ask anyone that's been married, has been in a long term relationship, or has ever had a new job. They will tell you that at some point, the honeymoon must end.

> Over the past ten years, I experienced a lot of moments in which I wanted to give up. Looking back, I'm appreciative of every step I made to stop talking about it and actually be about it.

I'm sure you've experienced a few honeymoons as well. Remember that time you started something new and were so excited about it? For the first couple of days, you felt invincible. You felt like nothing would get in your way. You were determined to succeed! You did everything you were supposed to do then WHAM! Suddenly, you got bored and wanted to revert to your old ways. Don't feel bad. You are not alone. Everyone has experienced that moment at some point in reaching their goals.

Once I realized the honeymoon phase was over, I knew it was time to get into the real work. So I added a healthy diet to my exercise routine. In addition to aerobics, I began walking a few times a week with friends. I joined so many gyms, tried different classes, and took a chance to try something new. I started to spend so much time in them that the workers knew me by name. Over the past ten years, I experienced a lot of moments in which I wanted to give up. Looking back, I'm appreciative of every step I made to stop talking about it and actually be about it.

We have all experienced moments of being TIRED of being tired. You know, those moments in which we feel like all hope is lost, and our cookie is crumbling. Those moments are called TURNING points. In those moments, our mind begins to replace every excuse with determination. It's in those moments that God is telling us it's time to make a change. Sometimes, we just don't know how to change. We don't know where to start. Now is the time! On the next page you will find a few questions to help you get started.

COOKIE BITES

1. Name a time you felt most uncomfortable in your skin.

2. How did that make you feel?

3. Without thinking about your weight, what would a perfect, healthy life look like for you? What would you do?

4

COOKIE DOUGH

WHAT WILL MOLD YOU INTO REACHING YOUR LIFETIME GOALS?

"Every day do something that will inch you closer to a better tomorrow." ~Doug Firebaugh

One day I went to an exercise boot camp class, and I thought, you know what? I would like to be an instructor. I wanted people to someday look at me and my journey, and say "If she did it, she can teach me and motivate me to do it."

I wasn't a size five like the girls that show up at most gyms. When I decided to get certified at the YMCA, I was probably a size 16. I wanted to do an exercise class for plus-sized women, but the plus-sized women were not showing up

– just the petite girls. There I was in my size sixteen sweats, instructing women that were a size two or three.

I taught at the YMCA for almost nine years. My classes were serious. You can ask anybody. Donna didn't play! My classes consisted of straight cardio and strength, similar to football training. I pushed people to the limit. "When you can't believe in yourself, I'm going to believe in you," I would say. "I believe in you. Give me just one hour for you." The people that are in my class often say, "Donna, it's not easy." But I knew

> My goal has never been to make people skinny. My goal is for them to empower themselves for a lifetime.

what it would take to get them to their goal. If it were easy, everyone would be doing it. This mindset separates those that want to live from those that just say they do. I wish somebody would have been hard on me. I'm not easy because I don't let people just come in and watch my class. If they just spectate they will tell themselves that they can't do it, but if they come in prepared to get dirty, I can push them the rest of the way!

My goal has never been to make people skinny. My goal is for them to empower themselves for a lifetime. My goal is to help them live and become healthy. That's what makes me different from many other trainers. I'm not just a trainer. I'm not a nutritionist. I'm a Healthy Lifestyle coach, I'm a motivator, and I let people know that. I tell them what has worked for me and what's worked for the girls that have been in my program. At the end of the class, once they have done lunges, squats, lifted weights, thrown medicine balls, pushed sleds, flipped over tires, and jumped rope (things they never imagined they could do) I look them in their eyes and say, "You did it. You should be proud of you. You're doing things that people wish that they could do. Move for the people that can't!"

I motivated everyone, even those slender size fives. Sure, they may be small, but they must be motivated too. It doesn't matter who you are! Besides, I was unaware of what was going on in their personal lives. Even though they appeared to be well put together outwardly, they could have been dealing with some real issues internally. Their husband could have divorced them two days ago, someone could have pissed them off, their kids might have just gotten on their last nerves, or they might even have health issues. We're all human. If you speak to the human condition, you will strike a chord with those that need to change their mindsets to lose weight and be healthy.

Revenge Is a Dish Best Served Cold

After I had lost about 40 pounds, I started going to D1 sports training. D1 is a facility that focuses on getting teens to the best D1 condition to get to the next level. They also have boot camp classes for adults. I had one-on-one sessions with a personal trainer. His name was Nate Bandy. On day one, he looked me straight in my face and said, "I'm going to push you! Just keep coming back!" Push me

Memories of my younger years motivated me to keep pushing... I can still hear my classmates howling with laughter as I attempted to throw myself into something that looked like a somersault.

he did. I enjoyed my one-on-ones; sometimes. At other times, I wanted to grab my water bottle and walk out the door. Actually once I did, and Nate was right there at my car telling me, "You can do this!"

Memories of my younger years motivated me to keep pushing. As a little girl, I was teased a lot because of my size. Each time I wanted to quit, a memory of the eight-year-old Donna played in my head. There was a particular incident that I remember like it was yesterday. It was my turn to do a somersault in class, and everybody was pointing at me and laughing. I was far from athletic! I can still hear my classmates howling with laughter as I attempted to throw myself into something that looked like a somersault. At D1, I felt like that kid again, but this time I was facing my biggest fear and finally becoming the athlete I'd always wanted to be.

I motivated myself by thinking of my growth. Sure, as a child, I wasn't picked to be on anyone's team. No one wanted "Fat Donna" on their team to play Tag, Hide and- Seek, or dodgeball, but now I'm doing relay races, climbing ladders, and flipping tires. They wouldn't pick me then, but I embraced the motto that success is the best revenge. I was determined to succeed.

Purpose Made Clear

I was asked to teach an exercise class in the inner city. It was in the middle of the summer, so you know it was hot! To put the icing on the cake, the facility had no air conditioner! That was enough to discourage anyone, but surprisingly, that didn't stop women from coming to class. They needed a change in their life and besides, the classes were free. Every day, more and more women came in determined and focused to achieve their goals. Even though they complained about aching and were mad because their hair was sweated out, I wanted them to understand that I believed in them. They griped and complained on Tuesday, but on Thursday they came right back for more.

My Rock

My Aunt Debra was another overweight person in my family. There were several, but people teased her too, so I felt she understood me. My Aunt Debra was very giving. She could cook just like my grandmother. She would make food for her family like nobody else could! She had four children, but when I visited her house I would get all of her attention because I was the youngest! I got any and everything I asked for. She truly loved me. She had a way of making me feel special. When we prepared meals together, Aunt Debra would always listen to me. I would go into her room some days and sit and talk to her about how people made me feel. She would always remind me that I was beautiful inside and out.

Everyone knew I was her favorite. She never judged me or talked about me for being overweight. She always used to say, "You are pretty." I felt like she was the only person in the world that understood and knew my struggles. I'll never forget the day I received the phone call that hospice was

> If you desire to do anything great or anything that could potentially change your life, you must identify your "why".

45

coming to get my aunt. She had been battling colon cancer for years, but we never thought it would get as bad as it did. The family was at her house every day visiting and helping where ever they could. I was so happy when I got some alone time with her. I told her that I'd lost weight and was helping women who struggled with weight like she and I had. In her weakened state, she looked at me and said, "Donna, do me a favor. When you help those women, please, talk to each one of them and take your time out to help them however you can. I want you to talk to each and every one of them, and you help them. Remember that you didn't have anyone to do that for you." With tears streaming down my face, I told her I would.

Find Your Why

Her words stuck with me. I remember vividly that no one told me why I should lose weight, why I should stick with it, and why I needed to do it for a lifetime. Aunt Debra's words gave me my "why". Her words tied purpose to my weight loss goals. Her words tied purpose to my life! If you desire to do anything great or anything that could potentially change your life, you must identify your "why". Your "why" is your reason for pushing through the hard times and the moments you feel like stopping. Your "why" will keep you focused on the goal. Without it, you're just going through the motions.

Dropping Nuggets

Now let's get back to that hot-box summer class. After each exercise class, I knew the ladies were tired and ready to jet out, but I sat cross and center, and I said, "You know what? You guys did a great job, but here is just one small tip." I wanted to hear their big or small weekly successes. Every day I would leave them with tiny little tips, little nuggets to take with them.

One of the tips might have been something like, "Drink eight glasses of water so you can feel better with your digestion." Then I gave what I called my "former fat girl" tips, like "Don't bring those sweets in your house. Why? Because you're going to smoke them!" They would all laugh. This was when I realized I had their ears. They sat around in a circle and listened. The class ended at eight, but I was there until after nine because everybody wanted to talk to me. They wanted to be heard. They wanted me to listen to their problems, so I did and still do. Everyone that sat in that big class of 65 at Carver Center had one thing in common: they needed help. Remember the women at the YMCA? They needed the same motivation as well. Both groups needed somebody to tell them that they were proud of them. That's exactly what I did. This was when I began to feel better about who I was and what I was doing. I realized that my journey was helping others, as well as myself.

Spending time with my clients gives me a sense of pride and makes me teary-eyed all at the same time. All I ever wanted was someone to tell me that they were proud of me. I may not have received this same type of love from other trainers, but it is such an honor to be able to be listening ears and an open heart to others.

COOKIE BITES

Aren't you sick of having those short, pointless weight loss goals? Lose weight for a birthday (gain it back), lose weight for a man (gain it back), or lose weight to get in that sexy dress (gain it back.) Everyone has their reasons for losing weight, but let's focus on lifetime changes instead of short, insignificant moments.

- (Ex.) Long-Term Motivation: I will eat better and exercise to live the best life, to feel better. My plan is to avoid diabetes, hypertension, or other hereditary illnesses.

- (Ex.) Short Term Motivation: I will live healthier to feel more confident in my clothes, be more active with my children, or motivate others.

Now think about your short term and long term motivation. What's going to keep you pushing well after the honeymoon phase is over?

1. What is your personal motivation to lose weight? (Dig deep. Remember the main reason should be you! Your friends and family can reap the benefits, but what will motivate you to be healthy for a lifetime?)

2. What has held you from reaching your lifetime goal?

3. How can you make yourself a priority?

4. List three small changes you can make every day that will last a LIFETIME. (Don't list anything major or unrealistic. Be honest with yourself!)

5. What will encourage you to invest in YOU for a lifetime? (Think of some ways to reward yourself along the way!)

What D.I.V.A.s are Saying...

I started Donna's D.I.V.A.s in November, 2012 so I could "lose some weight". Honestly, I never expected to lose the weight (because I never had before) and I never expected to last as long as I have. Two years later, I have lost some weight but I gained things far more important; confidence, strength and a sisterhood that I never felt before. I never imagined I would enjoy working out/exercising, but when you do it with people that support you, it's a great feeling. We are all shapes and sizes and no one casts any judgment, only encouragement. Donna is a fabulous leader, and our biggest supporter. I can't imagine doing this without all the fabulous women in our group.

Kelly

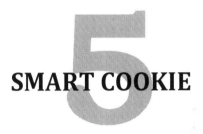

SMART COOKIE

YOU MUST CHANGE YOUR THINKING

Changing my relationship with food was like dealing with a bad break up. I didn't want to let go, but I had to. Just like a no-good ex, I could hear food saying, "Don't leave me!" "No, you've got to go, you have to get out of here!" I'd reply. It wouldn't be long before I was saying, "Oh, you're back again?" This cycle often repeated until I was tired of being sick and tired. I had to accept that my relationship with food was temporarily satisfying. Sure, it tasted great and got me through a lot of stressful situations, but it was detrimental to my health. From where I stood, it seemed like the good outweighed the bad in our relationship.

It's similar to being in a marriage that isn't meeting all of your needs. The bad or excess food wasn't meeting all of my needs and my potential for my life. It wasn't giving me the nourishment my body needed. I had to let it go. Now that

I've gotten out of the bad relationship, food and I can be respectable friends. We speak now and then, but before I feel like I'm reverting, I end the conversation and do something like running or working out to get food off my mind.

Even after you've decided to lose weight you may still encounter moments when you fall short. It's not about how many times you mess up; it's about the times you forgive yourself and kept pushing. You have to make up in your mind that no matter what happens, you will continue to push through. Don't just think it in your head, say it out loud! The words that come out of your mouth have the ability to build or tear down. Make sure the words that you speak over yourself and others are positive and uplifting.

> The words that come out of your mouth have the ability to build or tear down. Make sure the words that you speak over yourself and others are positive and uplifting.

Breaking the Cycle

You know what else pulled me through my weight loss journey? My relationship and connection to God. I had trainer after trainer after trainer. I had lost the weight, gained the weight, lost the weight, and gained the weight. Going up and down in my weight wore me out mentally and physically. I needed to do something a little different. I began praying in the morning, reading a scripture to get me through the day, and saying words of thanks every morning.

I read different books by Joyce Meyer and Joel Osteen. This led me to the Bible, and I realized that I could help other people through my process. For example, if you smile and people see it, it will make them smile; if you laugh and you're around people, it's contagious. God spoke to me and said, "I'm going to help you," and people started asking me to help them when they saw my transformation. I realized that my life wasn't my own anymore. It was a transformation right before people's eyes. My radio and TV audience, as well as my friends from social media, cheered on my progress. God had given me a gift of having a life again in my mid-twenties. If He can give me the gift of life again, after I had failed many times, then I could offer that gift of life to other women. Sometimes, our struggles aren't even for us. Sometimes, they are to help other people.

> There's nothing like recognizing your power and being brave enough to control and use it.

The more that I realized how God had my back, the more I had to say, "Donna, you've got something special." It was a gift of life for me. There's nothing like recognizing your power and being brave enough to control and use it.

There was a time when running three miles was a difficult task, now it's like second nature. I'm doing a marathon! Once I changed my mindset and told myself that I can and will be healthy, my lifestyle changed. I spoke over my life, and I asked others to speak positivity into my life. I envisioned what I wanted and I reached for it! Now, I'm doing half marathons, full marathons and I continue to push myself to do more. I am LIVING!! When I run, I talk to God. I use that time to say what I'm thankful for, what has hurt me or things that I may be angry about and just clear my head. I use that time to express my appreciation to move my limbs. Since I changed my mindset about life, I feel amazing! I feel alive! So many people take life for granted. We are all going through something. I had to channel my emotions towards a healthier future, despite what the present moment looked like. There are people in this world who wish that they could move and exercise, but they can't because they're paralyzed, sick, depressed or they have no limbs at all. I refuse to have functioning limbs and do nothing with them! Anytime I'm able to move around; I take the opportunity!

> I refuse to have functioning limbs and do nothing with them! Anytime I'm able to move around; I take the opportunity!

When people speak negatively about my weight loss, it motivates me. I've realized I can't please everyone. Just as food was once my go-to, being active is now everything to me. It reminds me that I am alive and well. This is the one thing no one can take from me because God gave me this amazing gift of life! I know that my life has been changed tremendously, because I now find pleasure in giving others what was never given to me. Each day that God breathes life into me, I take as an advantage to speak life into others. Changing your mind is half the battle. You have to wake up in the morning with expectancy. Know you are worth this journey. You have to believe you will emerge on the other side victorious! It is mind over matter. Start realizing that God loves you and has created a life for you to live daily. Look in the mirror NAKED and compliment yourself. Get on the scale, own the number. Yes, I know that seems extreme, but know that you can love who you are at this moment. You don't have to wait until you lose weight to love yourself and think positive. In fact, to change who you are, you must first change what you think about who you already are today.

COOKIE BITES

1. Name 5 things that you already love about yourself.
    1.

    2.

    3.

    4.

    5.

2. Perform an internet search on a new pair of gym shoes or workout clothes.

3. What home workouts could you do when you first wake up in the morning to start your day off in a positive way?

4. Ask three of your friends to list things they love about you. Have you ever noticed these things about yourself?

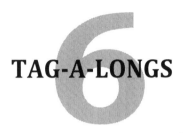

TAG-A-LONGS

I call my program, Donna's D.I.V.A.S, which stands for Determined Individuals Valuing Activities. My D.I.V.A.s program has a proven track record. It truly works. As the ladies walk through the door, I cheer them on. They can feel the positive energy before class even begins. These women are ready to reach their goals – they just need help doing it. My D.I.V.A.s come from different walks of life. They are real people, real women. When they start the program, they are at a range of sizes and have different strengths and weaknesses. I have small girls that run half marathons, but they may be missing something like upper body strength or confidence. Then I have women that are overweight, maybe in a size 24 just looking for somebody to say that they believe in them. In that class for one hour, I tell them, "We're not going back to who we used to be." I tell them this until they believe it!

I Encourage

I say everybody's name in my classes. "Good job, Sarah. Way to go, Kenya. Come on, Stephanie. Let's go, Crystal. Come on, Terri, let's get it!" I say those names. "Come on, Karen. Let's go, Kim. Come on! Let's go, Megan, you got it. Come on, Rebecca. Let's go, Emily."

Because those are the women that have been lost. Whether they are overweight, whether they are underweight, whether they just need the strength to move on. "Come on, Amy. Let's go Linda. Come on, Angie, you got it. Push yourself! Let's go, Patricia, I'm proud of you. High five! Let's go!" I say their names to remind them that this is about them and nobody else. I love on my girls during that hour even if they don't want to love themselves. For that one hour, I say their names and make them a priority because many of them won't get that after they leave my class. Many of them have to make others a priority. To feel alive for that one hour may just well be what they need to keep pushing through the next day.

> I say their names to remind them that this is about them and nobody else. I love on my girls during that hour even if they don't want to love themselves.

My goal in the D.I.V.A. program is to motivate 100,000 women nationwide to move for a lifetime. We have several locations, with awesome D.I.V.A. coaches. Not only do they workout consistently themselves, but they are also willing to share their personal stories and obstacles to motivate the beautiful women in their classes.

It's More Than Exercise and Eating Right

At the end of our class, we have D.I.V.A. Circle. During D.I.V.A circle, we share our D.I.V.A. success stories. We take a couple of minutes while we're stretching, and I ask them, "What is your biggest success story this week?" That success could be something like, "I was at the office, there were donuts on the counter and instead of eating a whole one, I ate a half one. I split it with somebody." Or "Right now instead of taking the elevator, I'm walking the steps."

> These stories remind me of the importance of having a support group. Sometimes it's the little, bitty, small successes we have during the week that no one cheers us on for.

Maybe it was, "Oh my goodness, I'm able to fit in smaller pants or I can finally zip my old pants up."

I've heard so many different success stories, and I'm wowed every time! One woman lives near a farm, and she shared, "Before, I wasn't able to lift the chicken feed, but now I can!" Another young lady once shared, "I just had a baby, and I can actually lift the carrier without being out of breath when I take my daughter into a restaurant." There was one success story that blew my mind. I'll never forget – one day, a lady raised her hand in the circle and said, "About a month and a half ago I was confined to a bed and breathing from an oxygen tank. Now I can come to your class. I feel amazing." It's stories like these that keep me going. These stories remind me of the importance of having a support group. Sometimes it's the little, bitty, small successes we have during the week that no one cheers us on for. D.I.V.A. circle is the time for everyone with a success story to be celebrated, or anyone with an issue to be uplifted.

Without my D.I.V.A.s, I wouldn't have achieved my weight loss goal. To me, the top D.I.V.A. is and will always be my mother. My mother has been in my classes from the start! We even workout together! Just to see my mom motivate and push herself after all of these years is amazing to me. There are twenty year-olds that won't even try what my mother doing!! I'm so proud of her! What I appreciate most is that she always reminds me, "Donna, you can do this!" My mom lost nearly a hundred pounds. To see her happy in her skin and motivated to continue going makes my heart sing.

> Each person that I have spoken with has been a motivation to my life. Hearing their personal stories have kept me inspired.

From Chattanooga to Birmingham, to Nashville, to Huntsville, and other D.I.V.A. locations I have realized that each of us are all going through something. It never fails, I can talk to a woman in our D.I.V.A. program in Chattanooga and talk to someone different in another city and the stories are so similar. We all could struggle through the same things, the same obstacles, and the same beast of not putting ourselves first and over compensating for everyone else. Each person that I have spoken with has been a motivation to my life. Hearing their personal stories have kept me inspired. There are several women in the program that were at home, taking care of their families with no personal

> Build a team, but remain the captain of your life!

reasons to enjoy life. It's a wonderful feeling to see women that once carried diseases (like cancer survivors), women, who were on blood pressure medicine, and women that were diabetic be empowered to take advantage of their lives means everything to me.

Gaining a Team!

I realized early in my journey I needed a support team. I needed to know I wasn't alone. When you begin to change your life, you may lose friends along the journey. Some friends may believe you are losing too much weight or you are obsessed with weight loss, simply because they aren't doing it or feel like they can't do it. Like I've heard before, some people can't go everywhere with you! At first, I wondered why I was ridiculed for doing something positive, but I then remembered what God spoke to me: "I will place friends in your life that will have your same interests along the way!" That He did! I have found wonderful workout partners, motivators and encouragers though the D.I.V.A.s program.

Sometimes we feel like we are alone on our journey, but we are not. Ultimately, it is you that will motivate you, but we all need people to surround us and motivate us! So how do you get them? Start by joining a walking/running team, a consistent workout class like D.I.V.A.s (hint, hint), or creating a team of like-minded individuals. But here is the key, never depend on anyone but yourself! At the end of the day, this is your journey. When I first started almost ten years ago, everyone wanted to do it. Now, there are only a few left. My mindset is "I can do all things through Christ who strengths me!" I remind myself often that what I do today will determine my tomorrow. That should be your mindset as well. Build a team, but remain the captain of your life! Get with people to exchange recipes or cooking tips. Involve your entire family. Make it fun!

COOKIE BITES

1. What workout program should you join? Or start? Who will you invite? What type of team do you need?

2. Who will be your team players?

3. How will you include your family and friends?

4. What will keep you motivated to stay on your journey?

5. Think of a positive motto to keep yourself motivated.

What D.I.V.A.s are Saying...

Before I started with Donna's D.I.V.A.S in July 2015, I was in "okay" health. I thought that if I worked out a few days a week, I could continue to eat whatever I wanted to. I quickly learned how nutrition impacted my lifestyle. Donna's workouts are by no means "easy", but it worth every minute.

Donna has taught me that my relationship with food is what I make of it. I learned that each food group has a significant importance; it's about moderation, instead of elimination. Before, I would eliminate a food group (carbs), in efforts to lose weight. This was ineffective for long term goals. I also learned how to avoid relapse eating on "comfort" foods during stressful times. Like any food addict, I was an emotional eater. Through Donna's D.I.V.A.S, I became more accountable of what I put into my body. I learned to replace the thought of a "diet" with the demonstration of a "lifestyle" change.

Cassie

7

YOU'RE NOT PERFECT, AND THAT'S OKAY!

Even though I lost a lot of weight, my body still has not been perfect. Women see my excess loose skin and say "Okay, Donna. I want to lose weight, but I don't want the flabby skin!" My response is and will always be the same, "Okay, would you rather be unhealthy or would you rather have a flawless body?" I feel like the loose skin is nothing compared to the weight that once kept me bound. Sure, I've thought about surgery. Do I want to do it? No, I don't. I love who I am. My body is imperfect, and it's okay. When I teach, I wear a sleeveless tank top. I don't mind that my arms are swinging everywhere. My excess skin says to everyone, "Sure, I used to be 300 pounds, but look at me now! I'm boxing. I'm punching. I'm living life. I'm not going to let a little skin stop me."

For some women, it may not be extra skin. It might be a scar, stretch marks, or a burn. No matter your imperfection may, you are still beautiful!

Here is something else I haven't been able to understand yet! So many of my ebony sistas won't work out because they don't want to sweat out their hair. Right now, at this moment, you must make a declaration that you won't let allow anything to stop you from becoming the best you that you can be! You can't let anything stop you from living your best life possible. It doesn't make sense to sit in a beauty salon for hours just to look beautiful while you're shaving years off your life with unhealthy living habits.

> It doesn't make sense to sit in a beauty salon for hours just to look beautiful while you're shaving years off your life with unhealthy living habits!

For so many years, the pain of being teased made me question who I was. It made me unhappy. I was so bitter that any time I tried to lose weight, I found myself thinking of how I was going to prove everyone from my past wrong, rather than proving myself right. I struggled with who I was. In public, I tried to be someone that everyone would like. I tried to hide behind my loud laugh and bright smile. When I got home (where it was just me and the cookies I prepared to smoke) I was unhappy. I beat myself up about being overweight. Would you believe I was in my twenties still depressed about things people said to me when I was in elementary school? I realized that I had to identify who I was. For so long, I didn't want anyone to see me because I didn't even realize who they were looking at. I wanted people to love me for me, but in actuality I didn't even love or know who I was.

We beat ourselves up so much. Often we revert to that kid again, or that failure we told ourselves we were. Forgiveness is important, not just of other people, but ourselves. When you make mistakes, don't give up! Move on! If you have a slice of cake or don't hit the gym, shake it off and accept the new day God has given you! You are worth it!! Demand your POWER BACK!!

COOKIE BITES

1. Did someone hurt you? Who should you forgive? How will you move on from it?

2. Have you failed your diet? Have you gained weight back before? What happened? Let's get your Power back!!

3. Imagine the new you! Some people have a vision board! When was the last time you saw yourself as what you wanted to be? Imagine yourself in grade school. On a separate sheet of paper or poster board, draw a picture of you now, then draw how you would like to look. Hang it up in a conspicuous place as a daily goal reminder.

4. Describe the new you. (Do not add people, just focus on you!)

POWER STEPS TO KEEP WEIGHT OFF FOR A LIFETIME

1. What you start you must continue
Just like a relationship we want people to keep up what they begin! And ladies you know we expect those roses every day. Yeah right. Be care of eliminating every food, working out six days a week, or starving yourself! Why? For example, if you eliminate bread and you visit an aunt and she cooks your favorite rolls you will crash and burn. Or if you start out working out 7 days a week, that's not realistic. Too many things come up. Create a Lifestyle eating regimen, workout regimen that you can see yourself doing 5 years from now.

2. Change your mindset with positive self-talk
Having a positive attitude will help your motivation. Before you walk into the gym, a class or when you begin your journey you need to know you are worth it! If you say you hate running, working out or eating better then you will get negative results.

3. Motivate yourself and others
When we typically start we tend to need someone to go for workouts with us or start a new diet with us and that's ok. But know if someone falls off from your group or workout you have to continue motivating yourself and find new people or groups to workout with or new people to motivate. Holding yourself accountable instead of depending on other is very important. Motivating others will keep you excited.

4. Eat in moderation instead of elimination

There are so many diets out; Atkins, gluten free, cabbage diet, protein only, etc. They all can work for weight loss but you need to keep the weight off. Be realistic with yourself. If you eat extreme and eliminate everything you can crash and burn. Plan to make healthy choices and eat what you enjoy in moderation. Instead of 2 pork chops, try one, love French fries, how about baking them? Instead of seconds how about one plate of things you love?

5. PUSH away from the table

Diet is majority of weight loss. Eating too many calories could result to weight gain. Knowing what you eat daily is essential to starting your weight loss journey. In order to lose and maintain write calories or log them into an app. My favorite is my fitness pal. Or weight watcher is an awesome way to begin. Working out is awesome but the scale will not change if you don't control what you eat once you have lost weight!

6. Weighing weekly

Many people say don't focus on the scale but if you have had a food addiction the scale can motivate you. Get on the scale, embrace your initial number and get angry, and know that you have the Power to change it!

7. Write down your goals
How can you get in the car if you don't know where you are going? Have a plan for both small and short term goals. Since this is for a lifetime keep up with goals every year. Whether it be to lose 5lbs, become more toned, or run faster.

8. Keep a regular exercise routine
Your goal should be to workout 3-5 days a week for life! Not temporary! Try different workouts; aerobics, circuit training, D.I.V.A.s classes, spin. Change your mindset and have fun!

9. Sign Up for Activities around health
There are several 5ks, walk/run, healthy eating classes, or even group workouts you should participate in. This will give you something to work up to. This will keep you motivated and a reason to train!

10. Love who you are
Having a positive attitude and believing in yourself is the best thing to stay healthy! Yes, the losing is important but regardless of your size you should believe in yourself.

11. Have support
You need friends and family for support. A team always works! Make it fun. Have walking groups. Start an eating healthy inbox or support team.

What
D.I.V.A.s
Are
Saying

I have worked out with the D.I.V.A.s for 3 years now. At my heaviest I was 244 lbs. I ate whatever I wanted when I wanted until one day I decided I wanted to feel better. I started weight watchers with two of my closest friends and one of them introduced me to the D.I.V.A.s group. Being a part of the group has changed my life. I don't think I would have made it as far as I have without these ladies.

Over the past 3 years, I have lost over 50 lbs. being a part of this group has given me strength and confidence. I am now one of the ladies who cheer others ladies on and encourage them to push through. When I first begin working out, the hardest thing for me was finding the time and motivation. The ladies in this group motivate me to get it in. My biggest accomplishment while being a part of the D.I.V.A.s was running my first half marathon this year along with 15 other D.I.V.A.'s! I am proud to be a part if this group!

Laquinta

I have always struggled with working out regularly. I would be challenged with staying motivated and to push myself to actually work out hard. I never felt proud of myself after a workout. I first met Donna outside of Donna 's D.I.V.A.s at an aerobics class she was teaching. I had not worked out in several months and was about 10 pounds overweight. Within minutes of the class starting, I started to have fun and let go of my insecurities. I loved her class so much, that I was compelled to talk to her afterwards. She invited me to come and try one of her Donna 's D.I.V.A.s classes.

The next week, I walked into a Donna 's D.I.V.A.s class. There were women of all shapes, ages and sizes and all ability levels. Right away, Donna reeled us in with her enthusiasm and her belief that we are all capable of being successful. I couldn't believe what I was doing.... pushups, squats, sprints, tire flips, bear crawls! I've always wanted to be one of "those people". We all were doing it. When I left her class that first night, I was proud of myself. I knew right away that this was I place where I belong. I am so grateful to be a part of this amazing group of women. I don't always sign up for each session, but now I work out regularly and I am able to motivate and push myself. I am strong. I am a D.I.V.A. You deserve this. Sign up today.

Kate

A little over a year ago I knew I needed to change, I was overweight and miserable. Donna's D.I.V.A.s was just the class I was looking for. Donna is great! The class is challenging for everyone at any level. It is so nice to have an instructor that knows her class individually, she knows when each of us are struggling, slacken or on it. She knows exactly how to motivate us, at times tough love but its Donna love. You earn very compliment with Donna and it is one of the best feeling when she yells out "I see you!" during class. She makes you want to be healthier and stronger seeing her walk the walk.

And you can't forget the D.I.V.A.s. They are so supportive in your journey. Having these ladies in class cheering you on makes you push through the pain. We laugh, sweat and have fun together! It's like having your own little fan club. I would have never lost 40lbs, ran a half marathon and felt great about myself if it wasn't for Donna and the D.I.V.A.s! Because of Donna and her D.I.V.A.s, I want and strive to be healthier and stronger for myself, my family and them. Even my husband is happy I joined the class and thinks it is one of the best decisions I made.

Peggy Sue

D.I.V.A.'S is everything to me! D.I.V.A.'S is motivating! D.I.V.A.'S helps you gain that confidence that you thought you lost! D.I.V.A.'S is A sister hood! I started D.I.V.A.'S in 2012 and it was life changing. D.I.V.A.'S is a lifestyle change, without D.I.V.A.'S I would not be who I am at this moment. Every time I wanted to give up it was always that voice telling me I can do it and reminding me of my personal goal. Knowing that there is someone that has been through what you are going through and can relate to you makes it that much better. D.I.V.A.'S will never give up on you, even when you feel like you have given up on yourself, there is always somewhere there for you!

Shantel

I joined my first D.I.V.A.s class in 2011 and I'm so glad I did. This was one of the best groups of ladies to workout with. Donna Elle is one of the most caring Trainers I have ever worked with it. She believes in you even when you don't believe in yourself. If it wasn't for Donna and the D.I.V.As, I would not have been able to run my half marathon. These ladies are so motivating and encouraging. I never knew that when I joined that session in January 2011, I would have made some life-long friends to help me through this life-long journey of becoming a healthier me. Go D.I.V.A.s!!!!!!!!

Patrice

I've done some form of exercising all of my adult life, but my journey with Donna's D.I.V.A.s has been a-mazing! It started 2 years ago this month and I have gained more than I have lost! I've gained strength, courage, confidence, and a new set of supportive D.I.V.A.s! And... a special friend, Donna, who is as beautiful as her smile! She is a no-non-sense motivator and trainer... I never thought I could last this long, but she keeps me going and I can always hear her say, "Don't cheat yourself"!

Rosie

Being a part of Donna's D.I.V.A.'s has helped us go further and pushed us to do more on our journey. Although we are doing this together as sisters it is great to have a group of ladies like the D.I.V.A.'s who uplift and support us on this journey. Since becoming a part of this class we workout more, we have completed several 5 & 10 k's and even took on the challenge of completing not one but two half marathons. Eating right & exercising has become a way of life. Donna encourages us by reminding us on how far we've come and not dwell on how far we have to go. She tells us to set healthy and realistic goals. Donna is very personable and open about her journey and is there to listen which helps us know we can do it. It's beneficial to us because there are other women who can relate and it has helped us to lose a total of 155 lbs. together. It is also beneficial because we get to help other women on their journey. This is a lifetime journey and not every day will be easy or go as planned. Remember if you fall off, don't beat yourself up, and just get back on track. It is truly worth it!!

Shenikia Sturnes & Robin Sturnes

I have worked out with the D.I.V.A.s for 3 years now. At my heaviest I was 244 lbs. I ate whatever I wanted when I wanted until one day I decided I wanted to feel better. I started weight watchers with two of my closest friends and one of them introduced me to the D.I.V.A.s group. Being a part of the group has changed my life. I don't think I would have made it as far as I have without these ladies.

Over the past 3 years, I have lost over 50 lbs. being a part of this group has given me strength and confidence. I am now one of the ladies who cheer others ladies on and encourage them to push through. When I first begin working

out, the hardest thing for me was finding the time and motivation. The ladies in this group motivate me to get it in. My biggest accomplishment while being a part of the D.I.V.A.s was running my first half marathon this year along with 15 other D.I.V.A.s! I am proud to be a part if this group!
Hope

"Sometimes being a "Donna's D.I.V.A." has nothing to do with fitness and everything to do with being healthy in all areas of your life. I personally have been inspired by Donna Elle's relentless, purpose-driven effort to shine light on the reality that for many women our physical health issues are in direct relationship to our mental, spiritual, and emotional status. Through countless hours of empowerment counseling and inspirational coaching, Donna Elle "The Ultimate D.I.V.A." has impacted my life in such a positive way that both my personal and professional life will never be the same. I encourage every woman in the nation to connect to the lifeline that is "Donna's D.I.V.A.s", you will never be the same.
Lakweshia

Made in the USA
San Bernardino, CA
18 March 2017